Table of Contents

Introduction

The point of "The Biggest Loser" tv display is to lose large amounts of weight as rapid as possible, through both a low-calorie food regimen and a lot of exercise. This makes for exquisite TV, however outside the strictly regulated environment of the Biggest Loser Ranch, it may not be as effective.

What Is the Biggest Loser Diet?

Like many other weight loss diets, the Biggest Loser diet is a low calorie eating program. It additionally stresses normal exercise.

Its meal plans provide 1,200–1,500 calories per day and include three meals, plus 2–three snacks from whole foods. The diet`s guidebook claims that ingesting frequently helps hold you full, balances your hormone levels, and provides power for normal exercise.

You`re meant to plan and prepare dinner dinner most meals on your own, cautiously counting calories and weighing and measuring foods. You`re similarly encouraged to hold a day by day meals log or journal.

How does it work?

For a safe 1–2 pounds (0. 5–0. 9 kg) of weight loss each week, subtract 500–1,000 calories from the number of daily calories you`re currently eating and use that as your initial calorie goal. The diet stipulates that 45% of your daily calories come from carbs like vegetables, fruits, and whole grains, 30% from dairy and animal or plant protein, and 25% from healthy fats like nuts, seeds, and olive oil, as well as sugar-free or low sugar desserts.

 three daily servings of protein from lean meats and fish, legumes, tofu and other soy foods, and low fat dairy products up to 200 daily calories from "extras," which include healthy fats, as well as treats and desserts

Day 1: Oatmeal with berries and low-fat milk; chicken breast with green salad and whole-grain bread; strawberries; tofu and veggie stir-fry; low-fat yogurt   Day 2: Egg white scrambled with spinach; brown rice, steak, and broccoli; low-fat cottage cheese; sole with asparagus and quinoa; apple with nut butter   Day 3: Whole-grain cereal with low-fat milk; green salad with turkey breast; carrot sticks with hummus; pork tenderloin with brown rice and green beans; melon   Day 4: Oatmeal with peaches and low-fat milk; whole-grain noodles with tomato sauce and turkey meatballs; whole-grain bread with nut butter;

tilapia and kale; raspberries Day 5: Egg white scrambled with green peppers; chicken breast with green salad and whole-grain bread; low-fat yogurt; tofu with brown rice and cauliflower; apple Day 7: Egg white scrambled with spinach; steak with green beans; whole-grain bread with nut butter; chicken breast with whole-grain noodles and peas; pear

Does it aid weight loss?

However, you shouldn`t expect the same results as the previous television show participants, who lost an average of 128 pounds (58 kg) over 30 weeks.

Various weight loss studies lasting 10–52 weeks indicate that low calorie diets result in an average weight loss of 22 pounds (9. 9 kg) from diet alone. Those who add exercise experience a whopping 29 pounds (13 kg) of weight loss, on average.

In a yearlong study in 7,285 people comparing various diets, including the Biggest Loser diet, low fat and low carb eating patterns result in slightly more weight loss than moderate macronutrient diets.

Other potential benefits

The Biggest Loser diet may have a few other benefits.

First, it may help you become a healthier eater because it incorporates whole, nutrient-dense foods and skips junk and fast food. It also stresses the importance of reading labels, measuring portion sizes, and keeping a food journal.

Using the Biggest Loser food pyramid to plan meals and snacks may likewise improve your diet quality. Researchers found this to be true for Americans who used the USDA's food pyramid to plan meals.

In fact, it may even reduce your cravings.

An analysis of 9 studies revealed that after 12 weeks, people who stuck to a low calorie diet had fewer cravings overall — and fewer specific hankerings for sweets, starches, and high fat foods.

 Other potential benefits

The Biggest Loser diet may have a few other benefits.

First, it may help you become a healthier eater because it incorporates whole, nutrient-dense foods and skips junk and fast food. It also stresses the importance of reading labels, measuring portion sizes, and keeping a food journal.

Using the Biggest Loser food pyramid to plan meals

and snacks may likewise improve your diet quality.

Researchers found this to be true for Americans

who used the USDA's food pyramid to plan meals.

In fact, it may even reduce your cravings.

An analysis of 9 studies revealed that after 12

weeks, people who stuck to a low calorie diet had

fewer cravings overall — and fewer specific

hankerings for sweets, starches, and high fat foods.

Foods to eat and avoid

This Biggest Loser diet emphasizes a variety of fresh, whole foods. Because few — if any — whole foods are banned and no foods are required, the plan is also flexible if you have dietary restrictions.

Fruits, non-starchy vegetables, and minimally processed whole grains will fill most of your plate. Starchy vegetables like sweet potatoes or squash are limited to just once or twice per week.

Protein choices include skinless poultry, leaner cuts of beef like sirloin or tenderloin, and seafood.

Fattier fish, such as salmon and sardines, are encouraged for their omega-3 fats, but remember that they're higher in calories than lean fish.

Vegetarian protein options include all legumes, plus soy products like tofu and tempeh. Egg whites and low fat or fat-free dairy products, including milk, nonfat yogurt, and low fat cheese, are also recommended sources of protein.

You're meant to limit nuts, seeds, avocados, oils, and other high fat foods to only 100 calories per day.

The diet's only other limited foods are sweets, snack treats, and alcohol, which are restricted to 100 calories per day. In fact, you're encouraged to skip these extras and instead allocate the 100 calories to healthy food choices.

Fruits and Vegetables

Four daily servings of fruits and vegetables are permitted, which could include:

- Carrots

- Greens

- Asparagus

- Cucumbers

- Apples

- Berries

- Melons

Whole Grains

This diet limits carbs and calories by reducing whole grains to two servings per day.

- Oatmeal

- Whole grain bread products

- Brown rice

- Quinoa

- Farro

Low-Fat Diary

The Biggest Loser Diet allows low-fat versions of dairy products, including:

- Cottage cheese

- Yogurt

- Sour cream

- Kefir

- Lean Protein

Three servings of lean protein per day are included

in the Biggest Loser Diet

- Sirloin steak

- Pork tenderloin

- Skinless chicken breast

- White fish

- Tofu

What You Cannot Eat

The Biggest Loser Diet is calorie-controlled. For that reason, certain foods are avoided.

Refined Grains

Whole grains serve up more nutrients and fiber than refined carbohydrates, so refined carbs are not included in the diet.

White bread products

White rice

Refined cereals and crackers

Caffeine

The Biggest Loser diet recommends avoiding caffeine completely. Since it can increase heart rate, caffeine doesn't pair well with strenuous exercise.

- Coffee

- Chocolate

- Soda

- Black tea

sample menu for 1 day

Here is a 1,500 calorie menu for 1 day on the Biggest Loser diet.

Breakfast

1 whole grain toaster waffle with 1 tablespoon of fruit spread and 1 cup (123 grams) of raspberries

1 poached or boiled egg

1 cup (240 mL) of fat-free milk

Snack

2 ounces (57 grams) of smoked salmon

2 Wasa crackers (or a similar multigrain crispbread)

Lunch

1 small whole grain tortilla with 3 ounces (85 grams) of roast beef, 1 tablespoon of horseradish, lettuce, and 3 thin slices of avocado

1 cup (150 grams) of seedless grapes

water or unsweetened iced tea

Snack

2 low fat mozzarella cheese sticks

1 large orange

Dinner

1 cup (240 mL) of fat-free lentil soup

1 serving of quinoa tabbouleh with tomato and

cucumber

3/4 cup (128 grams) of sliced melon

unsweetened tea

How to prepare the Biggest Loser Diet

Eating several times throughout the day may help you feel more full. The Biggest Loser diet allows for three meals and two snacks per day. The portions are small, but each meal or snack should contain protein and/or fiber to help defeat hunger. If you have a particular dietary need, such as vegetarian or gluten-free, it's relatively easy to adapt the Biggest Loser diet to work for you.

As for exercise, the TV show has participants performing vigorous exercise for three hours per day, including cardiovascular and strength training, under the supervision of fitness experts. This level of activity is not likely to be possible for most people and is likely to lead to overtraining, especially when combined with a low-calorie diet.

The at-home program features workout videos by the Biggest Loser trainers and instructions for beginning a workout program with as few as two training sessions per week at first. You can perform exercise at home or in the gym. There is also an optional run-walk program to follow that can help you train for a 5K or 10K race.

Although the Biggest Loser diet may be too low in calories for many people, it does have some components that may improve overall health.

Nutrition: This diet includes all major food groups, and its 4-3-2-1 pyramid may help users shift their daily menus to a healthier mix.

Resources: No special foods are required, but help in following this diet is readily available. The Biggest Loser Resort has a website with recipes and tips, and you can find books, cookbooks, food journals, exercise videos, and fitness equipment for sale. You can even watch old episodes of the TV

show if you find that motivating. But you also don't

have to use these tools if you don't feel they

benefit you.

Exercise: The need for exercise sets this diet apart

from many others. The Biggest Loser books suggest

following the diet for six weeks and including

exercise plans for those six weeks.

May meet daily nutrient needs: The Biggest Loser

diet does not cut out any major foods or food

groups. Everything is included, so with careful

planning (to account for portion size and calorie

count), those on this diet should be able to get the nutrients they need. This will mean choosing nutrient-dense foods, like whole grains, lean proteins, and vegetables.

May improve body composition: Since the Biggest Loser diet emphasizes protein and includes strength training, it may help preserve muscle often lost during low-calorie weight-loss diets. Improved body composition may help prevent health conditions and all-cause mortality.

One of the biggest pros of the Biggest Loser diet is that it can deliver short term results, especially if you have a lot of weight you want to get rid of. The 30-Day Jump Start can make a big difference, but for sustainable weight loss, the 6 weeks plan is even better.

Healthy in the Long Run

Nutritionally sound, the Biggest Loser diet is heart-healthy and can also help prevent and control diabetes. Since it also places a lot of importance on exercise, this diet plan is actually a healthy lifestyle that can also reduce the risk of cancer.

No Major Restrictions

If you're not a fan of diets that write off entire food groups, you'll be glad to know that one of the pros of the Biggest Loser diet is the fact that nothing is completely off limits. The guidelines in all the Biggest Loser diet books advise you to keep treats like desserts and alcohol to under 200 calories per day.

High Convenience

After you get used to the Biggest Loser diet pyramid, you won't run into a lot of trouble when you want to eat out, so the weight loss plan can be convenient. However, you'll still have to do some cooking yourself.

Plenty of Recipes and Resources

Besides the main books, you can also purchase recipe books, but one of the biggest pros of the Biggest Loser diet is the fact that you can also find plenty of recipes online, without any membership fees to a single site.

Cons of the Biggest Loser Diet

The Biggest Loser diet recommends extreme calorie restriction and so leads to some health risks. For that reason, the diet isn't recommended.

Restrictive: Although there are no food groups completely eliminated from the Biggest Loser diet, the restrictive amount of calories and servings of certain food groups each day might make following this diet feel like deprivation. The 200-calorie allowance for "other" foods is quite small.

Requires strict exercise: While exercise is always a good idea, especially if you are trying to lose weight, this diet makes it a requirement. If you cannot exercise or are not ready to, this makes the Biggest Loser diet inaccessible for you.

May lead to weight regain: Especially as depicted on the TV show, the Biggest Loser diet would be very difficult to sustain due to its low-calorie levels.3 The franchise's resort stays, and the plans outlined in its books are also short-term solutions. But you could use the Biggest Loser diet to kick off a weight-loss plan and then modify it (by increasing

calories and fat) to make it a longer-term option.

Restricted calories and fat: Some Biggest Loser diet

menus total just 1100 calories per day, with only

12% to 16% of those calories from fat. Both of

these figures are low—probably too low to be

either healthy or sustainable, especially if you are

adding in a lot of exercise for the first time.

Lowered metabolism: Any time you lose weight,

your body needs fewer calories than it did at your

prior weight. So you have to get used to eating less

to maintain your weight. Sometimes, especially if

you lose weight quickly (as is the goal with this diet), it's easy to lapse and regain that weight right back.

May Be Difficult to Follow

Flexibility is a plus for many dieters, but for others it's also one of the cons of the Biggest Loser diet. Sticking to a calorie ceiling can be complicated for some, especially when you also have exercise to worry about.

Exercise Is a Must

With a guideline of at least 2 and a half hour of moderate intensity activity every week and muscle-strengthening exercise on top of that, the Biggest Loser diet wants to keep you moving. You can choose from a wide range of activities, from resistance training to pilates.

Results Aren't as Dramatic as on TV

One of the most obvious cons of the Biggest Loser diet is that the dieters who participate in the show are a lot more motivated than viewers. They also get access to experts who advise and encourage them, along with a biz prize as an incentive. You're less likely to experience the same dramatic results at home.

You'll Have to Count Calories

Since you're supposed to pay attention to calories, especially when it comes to treats, you'll have to do quite a lot of math on this diet, which isn't something every dieter is keen on doing.

While each book will set you back around $16, one of the cons of the Biggest Loser diet is that you'll end up spending more on groceries, especially fresh fruits and vegetables, along with fish and whole grains

Is the Biggest Loser Diet a Healthy Choice for You?

The Biggest Loser diet made for great drama on TV, but in real-life practice, it is a fairly simple concept that is similar to other weight-loss plans. Like other diets, the Biggest Loser diet creates a calorie deficit designed to bring on weight loss. Then it revs up that deficit with extra exercise.

The U.S. Department of Agriculture's Dietary Guidelines for Americans suggest getting a balanced diet of fruits, vegetables, grains, proteins, and low-fat dairy products.6 This is similar to the Biggest Loser diet's recommendations.

The USDA suggests a basic figure of 2000 calories per day for weight maintenance, although this number varies based on age, sex, weight, and activity level. For weight loss, the USDA suggests reducing calories from your maintenance amount based on your activity level. The Biggest Loser diet generally goes beyond that number. A healthier (but perhaps slower) way to lose weight is to use this calculator to determine your daily calorie need for weight loss.

How easy is the Biggest Loser Diet to follow?

Because the Biggest Loser diet doesn`t ban entire food groups, you shouldn't have trouble complying long-term. For instance, you can look to any of the cookbooks, including one for family dinners and another just for your sweet tooth. For those who don't think healthy meals are flavorful, there's also

Biggest Loser chef and dietitian Cheryl Forberg's

"Flavor First" cookbook. You'll find more free

Biggest Loser recipes online.

 You can eat out on the Biggest Loser diet. Figure

out what you want before you head out, and don't

let the tempting smells at the restaurant change

your mind. For an extra support boost, you can

hire a one-on-one coach or join the online

community for a fee. You shouldn't get too hungry

on the Biggest Loser diet.

The Biggest Loser diet can be tasty – or not.

.

How much should you exercise on the Biggest Loser Diet?

Exercise – aleven though broadly defined – is a key part of the Biggest Loser diet. If you`re following "6 Weeks to a Healthier You," each week drills home the importance of exercise in combating and reversing common weight-related conditions, from Type 2 diabetes to high blood stress and coronary heart disease. You'll begin out with body-weight training (lunges, squats, push-ups), then eventually move into aerobics, strength and resistance training, and even yoga and Pilates.

 What subjects most, though, is that you are moving. Adults are generally encouraged to get at least and a 1/2 of hours of moderate-depth activity (like brisk walking) a week, along side a couple days of muscle-strengthening activities. Find an activity that you love and appearance forward to doing whether it`s hula-hooping or hip hop dances classes. Make it fun.

7-Day Meal Plan

Monday

Breakfast:

half cup egg whites scrambled with 1 teaspoon olive oil, 1 teaspoon chopped basil, 1 teaspoon grated Parmesan, and half cup cherry tomatoes

1 slice whole-grain toast

half cup blueberries

1 cup skim milk

Snack:

half cup fats-loose Greek yogurt topped with 1/four cup sliced strawberries

Lunch:

Salad made with: three/four cup cooked bulgur, four oz. chopped grilled chook breast, 1 tablespoon shredded low-fat cheddar, diced grilled veggies (2 tablespoons onion, 1/four cup diced zucchini, half cup bell pepper), 1 teaspoon chopped cilantro, and 1 tablespoon low-fats vinaigrette.

Snack:

2 tablespoons hummus and 6 baby carrots

Dinner:

four oz. grilled salmon

1 cup wild rice with 1 tablespoon slivered toasted almonds

1 cup wilted child spinach with 1 teaspoon each olive oil, balsamic vinegar, and grated Parmesan

half cup diced cantaloupe crowned with

half cup all-fruit raspberry sorbet and 1 teaspoon chopped walnuts

Tuesday

Breakfast:

three/four cup steel-cut or old skool oatmeal prepared with water; stir in half cup skim milk

2 links country-fashion turkey sausage

1 cup blueberries

Snack:

half cup fat-free ricotta cheese with half cup raspberries and 1 tablespoon chopped pecans

Snack:

half cup fats-loose cottage cheese with half cup salsa

Dinner:

1 turkey burger

three/four cup roasted cauliflower and broccoli florets

three/four cup brown rice

1 cup spinach salad with 1 tablespoon light balsamic French dressing

Wednesday

Breakfast:

Omelet made with four egg whites and 1 complete egg, 1/four cup chopped broccoli, 2 tablespoons every fat-free refried beans, diced onion, diced mushrooms, and salsa

Quesadilla made with half of one small corn tortilla and 1 tablespoon low-fat jack cheese

half cup diced watermelon

Snack:

half cup fats-loose vanilla yogurt with 1 sliced apple and 1 tablespoon chopped walnuts

Lunch:

Salad made with 2 cups chopped Romaine, four ounces grilled chook, half cup chopped celery, half cup diced mushrooms, 2 tablespoons shredded low-fats cheddar, and 1 tablespoon low-fat Caesar dressing

1 medium nectarine

1 cup skim milk

Snack:

1 fat-free mozzarella string cheese stick

1 medium orange

Dinner:

four ounces shrimp, grilled or sauteed with 1 teaspoon olive oil and 1 teaspoon chopped garlic

1 medium artichoke, steamed

half cup complete wheat couscous with 2 tablespoons diced bell pepper, 1/four cup garbanzo beans, 1 teaspoon chopped sparkling cilantro, and 1 tablespoon fat-free honey mustard dressing

Thursday

Breakfast:

1 light whole-grain English muffin with 1 tablespoon nut butter and 1 tablespoon sugar-free fruit spread

1 wedge honeydew

1 cup skim milk

2 slices Canadian bacon

Snack:

Yogurt parfait made with 1 cup low-fat vanilla yogurt, 2 tablespoons sliced strawberries or raspberries, and 2 tablespoons low-fat granola

Lunch:

Wrap made with four oz. thinly sliced lean roast beef, 1 6-inch whole wheat tortilla, 1/four cup shredded lettuce, three medium tomato slices, 1 teaspoon horseradish, and 1 teaspoon Dijon mustard 1/2 cup pinto beans or lentils with 1 teaspoon chopped basil and 1 tablespoon light Caesar dressing

Snack:

8 baked corn chips with 2 tablespoons guacamole (try one of these guac recipes)

Dinner:

4 ounces grilled halibut

1/2 cup sliced mushrooms sauteed with 1 teaspoon olive oil, 1/4 cup chopped yellow onion, and 1 cup green beans

Salad made with 1 cup arugula, 1/2 cup halved cherry tomatoes, and 1 teaspoon balsamic vinaigrette

1/2 cup warm unsweetened applesauce with 1/4 cup fat-free vanilla yogurt,

1 tablespoon chopped pecans and dash cinnamon

Friday

Breakfast:

Burrito made with: 1 medium whole wheat tortilla, 4 scrambled egg whites, 1 teaspoon olive oil, 1/4 cup fat-free refried black beans, 2 tablespoons salsa, 2 tablespoons grated low-fat cheddar, and 1 teaspoon fresh cilantro

1 cup mixed melon

 Snack:

3 ounces sliced lean ham

1 medium apple

 Lunch:

Turkey burger

Salad made with: 1 cup baby spinach, 1/4 cup halved cherry tomatoes, 1/2 cup cooked lentils, 2 teaspoons grated Parmesan, and 1 tablespoon light Russian dressing

1 cup skim milk

Snack:

1 fat-free mozzarella string cheese stick

1 cup red grapes

Dinner:

5 ounces grilled wild salmon

1/2 cup brown or wild rice

2 cups mixed baby greens with 1 tablespoon low-fat Caesar dressing

1/2 cup all-fruit strawberry sorbet with 1 sliced pear

Saturday

Breakfast:

Frittata made with 3 large egg whites, 2 tablespoons diced bell peppers, 2 teaspoons chopped spinach, 2 tablespoons part-skim shredded mozzarella, and 2 teaspoons pesto 1/2 cup fresh raspberries

1 small bran muffin

1 cup skim milk

Snack:

1/2 cup low-fat vanilla yogurt with 1 tablespoon ground flaxseed and 1/2 cup diced pear

Lunch:

4 ounces sliced turkey breast

Tomato-cucumber salad made with 5 slices tomato, 1/4 cup sliced cucumber, 1 teaspoon fresh chopped thyme, and 1 tablespoon fat-free Italian dressing

1 medium orange

Snack:

Smoothie made with 3/4 cup skim milk, 1/2 banana, 1/2 cup low-fat yogurt, and 1/4 cup sliced strawberries

Dinner:

4 ounces red snapper baked with 1 teaspoon olive oil, 1 teaspoon lemon juice, and 1/2 teaspoon no-sodium seasoning

1 cup spaghetti squash with 1 teaspoon olive oil and 2 teaspoon grated Parmesan cheese

1 cup steamed green beans with 1 tablespoon slivered almonds

Sunday

Breakfast:

2 slices Canadian bacon

1 whole-grain toaster waffle with sugar-free fruit spread

3/4 cup berries

1 cup skim milk

Snack:

1/4 cup fat-free cottage cheese with 1/4 cup cherries and 1 tablespoon slivered almonds

Lunch:

Salad made with: 2 cups baby spinach, 4 ounces grilled chicken, 1 tablespoon chopped dried cranberries, 3 slices avocado, 1 tablespoon slivered walnuts, and 2 tablespoons low-fat vinaigrette

1 apple

1 cup skim milk

Snack:

1/4 cup plain fat-free Greek yogurt with 1 tablespoon sugar-free fruit spread and 1 tablespoon ground flaxseed

1/4 cup blueberries

Dinner:

4 ounces lean pork tenderloin stir-fried with onions, garlic, broccoli, and bell pepper

1/2 cup brown rice

5 medium tomato slices with 1 teaspoon each chopped ginger, chopped cilantro, light soy sauce, and rice wine vinegar

Recipes

Ham and cheese breakfast melt

Ingredients

- 1 Thomas' Light Whole Grain English Muffin, split

- slice (1 ounce) lean, low-sodium ham or lean Canadian bacon

- egg whites

- slice low-or reduced-fat Cheddar cheese Salt and pepper to taste

Instructions

1. Coat a ring with olive oil and cook an egg spray.

2. Toast the muffin halves until they're lightly browned. While the muffin toasts, warm the ham for about 1 minute in a small nonstick skillet. Remove the ham from the skillet and place it on half of the toasted English muffin. Cover to keep it warm.

3. Place the prepared egg ring in the nonstick skillet over medium heat. Pour the egg

whites into the ring. Cover the pan and cook over medium heat for about 3 minutes, or until the eggs are nearly set. Run a knife or spatula around the inside edge of the ring to break the egg loose. Remove the ring. Flip the egg over and cook it for about 30 seconds longer, or until done.

4. Place the egg on top of the ham. While the egg is piping hot, lay the cheese over it. Top with the remaining muffin half. Serve hot.

Ingredients:

- 1 head of fresh lettuce

- 1/3 cup olive oil (for dressing)

- 1 cucumber

- 4 tbsp lemon juice (for dressing)

- 2 fresh in-season tomatoes

- 1 tsp honey (for dressing)

- 1/4 red onion

- salt and pepper, to taste

- 1 bunch fresh basil

Directions:

1. For the salad: wash and dry the lettuce. Tear it into bite-size pieces. Peel the cucumber and cut it into bite-sized bits. Wash the tomatoes and cut them into bite sized pieces. Peel the onion and slice it as thin as possible. Wash and chop the basil into large pieces.

2. In a large mixing bowl, combine the lettuce, cucumbers, tomatoes, onions and basil. Toss together so the ingredients are well mixed.

3. For the dressing: place the dressing ingredients in a container with a tight-fitting

lid. Cover the container and shake vigorously.

4. Add the dressing to the salad, toss and serve immediately.

Biggest Loser Stew

Ingredients

- 1 tablespoon All purpose flour

- 1/8 teaspoon garlic powder

- 1/8 teaspoon Onion powder

- 1/8 teaspoon salt

- pinch Black pepper

- 1 lb round steak ; cut into cubes

- 2 teaspoon olive oil

- 1 teaspoon minced garlic

- 1 teaspoon Dried thyme

- 2 cans beef both

- 2 large carrots ; peeled and sliced

- 1 lb sweet potatoes ; peeled and cubed

Instructions

1. In a medium resealable plastic bag, combine the flour, garlic powder, onion powder, salt, and pepper. Add the beef and shake the bag until all the cubes are coated. Refrigerate for at least 15 minutes.

2. Set a large nonstick soup pot over medium-high heat until it is hot enough for a spritz of

water to sizzle on it. Add the oil. Brown beef and then cut into cubes.

3. Return beef to pot and reduce the heat to medium. Add the garlic, and thyme. Cook for about 1 minute more.

4. Add the broth and carrots. Increase the heat to high. When the broth comes to a boil, reduce the heat to low so the mixture simmers gently.

5. Cover and cook for 45 minutes.

6. Add the potatoes. Cook for another 45 minutes, or until the beef is fork tender.

7. Season with additional salt and pepper.

8. Serve your beef stew immediately.

Ingredients

- 2 pounds extra lean ground beef

- 1 teaspoon olive oil

- 1 red bell pepper (diced)

- 1 cup celery (chopped)

- 1/2 cup water chestnuts (sliced)

- 1 cup green onions

- 1 1/2 tablespoons fresh ginger root (finely grated)

- 3 cloves garlic

- 2 tablespoons soy sauce (use Gluten Free Soy Sauce if you are gluten free)

- 1/2 teaspoon red pepper flakes

- 2/3 cup hoisin sauce

- 1/4 cup sliced almonds

- lettuce (Head of your favorite, butter, iceburg, Romaine, ect)

Instructions

1. Wash the bell pepper, celery stalks, and green onions.

2. Using a sharp knife, cut the red bell pepper in half. Remove and discard the center of the bell pepper. Using a knife or a vegetable chopper, finely chop the red bell pepper into small pieces. Place the peppers into a small bowl.

3. Thinly slice 3-4 stalks of celery into slivers.
    Place the celery into the bowl with the red
    peppers.

4. Slice the green onion into small slivers,
    ensuring you use both the green and white
    part of the onion. Ensure you discard the
    bottom root part of the green onions.

5. Using a vegetable peeler, remove the
    peeling from the ginger and then finely chop
    using either a sharp knife or the vegetable
    chopper.

6. Next, remove the papery skin from the garlic
    and finely chop using either a knife or the
    vegetable chopper.

7. Drain the can of water chestnuts and chop into small pieces.

8. Place the green onions, ginger, garlic, and water chestnuts into a separate bowl.

9. At this point of the process, you should have 2 bowls; 1 bowl containing the chopped red bell peppers and celery and 1 bowl containing the chopped water chestnuts, garlic, ginger, and green onions.

10. Place a large skillet over medium-high heat and add 1 Tablespoon of extra-virgin olive oil. Once the oil has heated, sauté the red bell pepper and celery for 2-3 minutes.

11. Next, add the raw ground meat, sliced green onions, chopped ginger, red pepper flakes, garlic, and water chestnuts to the skillet with the red pepper and celery.

12. Cook the mixture over medium-high heat for 8 to 10 min, or until the meat is cooked all the way through, ensuring the meat is no longer pink.

13. Slowly stir in the soy sauce, hoisin sauce, and almonds with the meat and vegetable mixture until well combined. Once well combined, allow the mixture to simmer on medium-low heat for 5-7 minutes.

14. Scoop ¼ cup of the meat and vegetable mixture onto the leaf lettuce. Roll the lettuce like a wrap and enjoy!

Banana Breakfast Smoothie

Ingredients

- 1 banana (medium, sliced)

- 1 cup skim milk

- 3/4 cup nonfat vanilla yogurt

- 1/4 cup pineapple juice

- 1/2 tablespoon honey

Directions:

1. Add all ingredients to the blender. Process

    the bananas, milk, yogurt, juice and honey

    until

    smooth. Serve immediately.

Chicken Salad Sandwich

Ingredients

- 1 pound trimmed boneless, skinless chicken

  breasts

- 3 teaspoons extra-virgin olive oil

- Ground black pepper, to taste

- 3 tablespoons fat-free plain yogurt

- 3 tablespoons Dijon mustard

- 1/3 cup chopped celery

- 1/3 cup seedless grapes, each cut in half

- 1/3 cup chopped red apple

Preparation

2. Preheat a grill to high heat.

3. Rub the chicken all over with 1 teaspoon of the olive oil and season with salt and pepper.

4. Place on the grill and cook for 3 to 5 minutes per side, or until the chicken is no longer pink and juices run clear. Allow the chicken to cool, then cut it into bite-sized cubes.

5. In a large glass or plastic mixing bowl, whisk together the remaining 2 teaspoons olive oil, the yogurt and mustard.

6. Add the chicken, celery, grapes, and apple. Gently toss well to combine. Season with salt and pepper and serve.

BBQ Bacon Meatloaf

Ingredients

- 1lb ground turkey

- 4 slices of turkey bacon cut in half crosswise

- 1clove garlic chopped

- 1c chopped red onion

- 2 egg whites

- 2/3 cup oats

- 1/2 cup milk

- 1/3 cup BBQ sauce

Instructions

1. Preheat oven to 350

2. Spray loaf pan with Pam

3. heat the skillet on medium heat. Add onion and bacon. Cook for 6-8min. or until bacon is done and onions start to brown.

4. In a large bowl mix milk and oats. Let stand for 3 min.

5. Add cooled onion mixture, ground turkey, garlic and egg whites.

6. Mix with your hands and form into loaf.
   Place in a loaf pan and top with BBQ sauce.

7. Bake for 35-40min.

Baked Eggs in Turkey Cups

Ingredients

- 6 ounces deli turkey, very thinly sliced

- 3/4 cup salsa or grilled vegetables

- 18 large egg whites or 2 1/4 cups liquid egg
  white or egg substitute (see note below)

- 2 tablespoons fresh cilantro, chopped

- 2 tablespoons grated low-fat Cheddar
  cheese

Instructions

1. If Using fresh eggs: Separate 18 whites into a medium mixing bowl Add 1/2 teaspoon salt and whisk lightly.

2. Transfer to a liquid measuring cup. Let stand while you prepare the rest of the ingredients.

3. Preheat the oven to 400ºF. Lightly coat each cup of a standard-sized nonstick muffin pan with olive oil cooking spray.

4. Line each muffin cup with 1/2 ounce of the turkey. There will probably be a little excess extending from the top of each cup.

5. Spoon 1 tablespoon of the salsa or grilled vegetables into each cup.

6. Measure 3 tablespoons of the egg whites or egg substitute into each muffin cup. (After the first "muffin," you can pour the whites from the liquid measuring cup to the same level as the fist muffin cup, rather than measuring 3 tablespoons each time.)

7. Place the muffin pan in the oven and bake for 10 to 12 minutes, or until the eggs are puffed and the center is set.

8. Carefully remove the baked eggs from the pan and place 2 egg cups on each serving plate.

9. Garnish with the cilantro and cheese.

Oatmeal Pancakes

Ingredients

- 6 large egg

- 1 cup rolled oats, dry

- 1 cup cottage cheese (1% M.F.)

- 2 tsp granulated sugar

- 1 tsp cinnamon

- 1 tsp vanilla extract, imitation, without alcohol

Instructions

1. In a blender, blend all ingredients until smooth.

2. Heat a griddle or large non-stick skillet over medium-low heat.

3. Spray with non-stick cooking spray.

4. For each pancake pour 1/4 cup of batter on a griddle. Flip when they start to bubble.

5. Cook until golden brown.

6. Repeat with remaining batches, spraying the griddle as needed.

Greek Goddess Salad

Ingredients

- 3 tablespoons minced fresh parsley leaves

- 4 pitted kalamata olives1 clove garlic, minced

- 5 tablespoons Lemon Juice, to taste

- 1/2 med cucumber, seeded and chopped

- 1/2 med red or orange bell pepper, chopped

- 1 medium tomato, seeded and chopped

- 1/3 cup finely chopped red onion

- 1 ounce crumbled reduced-fat feta cheese

- 1 small grilled chicken breast, sliced.

Directions

1. In a serving bowl, combine the parsley olives,

    and garlic.

2. Whisk in 4 tablespoons lemon juice.

3. Add the cucumber, bell pepper, tomato,

    onion, and 3 tablespoons of the cheese.

4. Toss to coat the ingredients with the

    dressing.

5. Taste and add up to 1 tablespoon more

    lemon juice, if desired.

6. Scatter the chicken over the salad, if desired.

    Top with remaining cheese.

Sauteed peppered mushrooms

Ingredients

- 1 1/2 teaspoons extra-virgin olive oil

- 1 1/2 pounds sliced button mushrooms

- 1 tablespoon freshly minced garlic

- 1 tablespoon Worcestershire sauce

- 1/2 teaspoon ground pepper (freshly ground

  is possible)

- Salt, to taste

Directions

1. Makes 4 (about 3/4 cup) servings

2. This is very good!

Cranberry Oatmeal Muffins

Ingredients

BOWL ONE

- 2 cups rolled oats

- 2½ cups skim milk

- 1 cup unsweetened applesauce

- 1 cup dried cranberries

BOWL TWO

- 2 eggs beaten

- 2 cups splenda (you could substitute sugar)

- 4 teaspoons vanilla extract

- ⅔ cup canola oil

BOWL THREE

- 2½ cups whole wheat flour

- 3 teaspoons baking powder

- 1 teaspoon baking soda

- 2 teaspoons cinnamon

- 1⅓ cup chopped walnuts

- 1 teaspoon salt

Instructions

1. Preheat the oven to 375 degrees. Add bowl one to bowl two and mix well.

2. Add to bowl three and mix just enough to moisten (you don't want to overmix these!).

3. Fill muffin tins 2/3 full and bake for about 20 minutes.

4. To check and make sure they are done, insert a toothpick in a muffin and make sure that it comes out clean.

Turkey Chili

Ingredients

- 1 lb ground turkey extra lean

- 3 garlic cloves minced

- 2 medium onions finely chopped

- 3 large celery stalks chopped

- 2 medium bell peppers chopped

- 14 oz can low sodium red kidney beans drained & rinsed

- 14 oz can low sodium white beans drained & rinsed

- 28 oz can tomato sauce or crushed tomatoes low sodium

- 1 cup chicken or vegetable broth low sodium

- 1 tbsp chipotle pepper in adobo sauce minced

- 1 tbsp chili powder low sodium

- 1 tbsp taco seasoning low sodium

- Salt and ground black pepper to taste

- Oil for frying

- Lime, cilantro, cheese, yogurt, chips etc. for serving

Instructions

1. Preheat a large 5-6 quart Dutch oven, heavy bottom pot or ceramic non-stick skillet on high heat and add ground turkey. Cook until small pieces form or about 5 minutes, stirring and breaking into small pieces with spatula constantly. Transfer to a bowl or large slow cooker, and set aside.

2. Return the skillet or pot to medium heat and swirl a bit of oil to coat. Add garlic and onion, sauté until translucent or 5 minutes, stirring occasionally. Add celery and bell peppers, sauté for 5 more minutes, stirring

occasionally. If using a slow cooker, transfer there, or leave in a dutch oven.

3. Then add red kidney and white beans, tomato sauce, broth, chipotle pepper, chili powder, taco seasoning and pepper.

4. Cover, bring to a boil, reduce heat to low and simmer for about 30 minutes. In a slow cooker, cook on Low for 8 hours or on High for 4 hours.

5. Stir and adjust salt to taste, if necessary. Serve warm with your favorite toppings!

Ingredients

- 2 cups baby spinach leaves or coarsely chopped flat- leaf spinach, rinsed

- 1 tablespoon olive oil

- 1 cup diced red onion

- Pinch of salt

- 3 ounces cremini or button mushrooms, trimmed and sliced (about 1 cup)

- 1 small (about 3 ounces) russet potato, cut into 1/4- inch cubes (about 1/2 cup)

- 1/2 red bell pepper, cut into 1/4- inch cubes (about 3/4 cup)

- 4 large eggs

- 1/2 cup crumbled low- fat feta cheese

- 1 teaspoon chopped fresh oregano leaves

- 1/4 teaspoon ground black pepper

Instructions

1. Set a rack about 4 inches from the broiler and preheat the broiler to low.

2. Heat an 8- to 10- inch cast- iron or other ovenproof (not nonstick) skillet over low heat. Add the spinach with the rinse water still clinging to the leaves (if the spinach is completely dry, add a tablespoon of water to the pan with the spinach). Cover and cook

until the leaves have barely wilted, about 1 minute. Transfer to a colander and use tongs to squeeze out as much liquid as possible. Wipe the skillet clean.

3. Add the olive oil to the cleaned skillet and heat over medium heat. Add the onion and salt and cook, stirring occasionally, until the onion is beginning to soften, about 2 minutes. Add the mushrooms and cook, stirring occasionally, until lightly browned, about 2 minutes. Stir in the potato and pepper, cover, and cook, stirring once or twice, until the potato is tender but still firm, another 5 to 7 minutes.

4. Meanwhile, in a medium bowl, whisk the eggs until lightly beaten. Stir in the reserved spinach, the feta, oregano, and black pepper. When the potato mixture is cooked, evenly pour the egg mixture over it. Cook until the eggs are set around the edges, about 10 minutes.

5. Place the skillet under the broiler for 1 to 2 minutes, until the top of the frittata is puffed and lightly browned. Serve hot.

Ingredients

- Olive oil spray, for the grill pan

- 2 slices crusty whole- wheat bread, such as boule or country loaf

- 1 1/2 teaspoons Dijon mustard

- 1/4 teaspoon honey

- 1 1/2 ounces thinly sliced organic Black Forest or other smoked ham

- 1/2 ounce reduced- fat Cheddar cheese, thinly sliced

- 1/4 Granny Smith apple, cored and thinly sliced

- Freshly ground black pepper to taste

Instructions

1. Spray a grill pan with olive oil and heat over medium- high heat until hot but not smoking. Place the bread slices on the grill and grill until grill marks appear on both sides, about two minutes per side.

2. Meanwhile, in a small bowl, place the mustard and honey. Stir with a small spoon until well combined.

3. Place the grilled bread on a work surface and spread the mustard and honey mixture on both slices. On one slice of bread, place the ham, gently folding each slice in thirds to give the sandwich some height.

4. Arrange the cheese slices on top and then the apple slices. Grind some black pepper on the apple.

5. Place the other slice of grilled bread on top. Slice the sandwich in half. Serve.

Guacamole

Ingredients

- 2 plum tomatoes, finely chopped (about 1 cup)

- 1/4 cup finely chopped red onion

- 2 tablespoons fresh lime juice

- 2 tablespoons chopped fresh cilantro leaves

- 1/2 teaspoon seeded and minced fresh chiles

- 1/4 teaspoon salt

- 1/4 teaspoon ground cumin

- 2 small, ripe avocados, pitted and peeled

Instructions

1. In a medium bowl, gently integrate the tomatoes, onion, lime juice, cilantro, chiles, salt, and cumin. Stir.

2. Add the avocados and use a fork to gently mash and combine them with the different ingredients.

3. Guacamole is best served soon after preparation, however it can be stored in a tightly covered container in the fridge for up to two days.

Fancy Fish Sticks

Ingredients

- 11/2 pounds grouper (haddock or cod work well, too)
- cooking spray
- 1 Tbsp. fresh lime juice
- 1 Tbsp. fat-free mayonnaise
- 1/8 tsp. onion powder
- 1/8 tsp. freshly ground black pepper

- 1/2 cup fresh breadcrumbs

- 11/2 Tbsp. melted Smart Start

- 2 Tbsp. chopped fresh parsley

Instructions

1. Preheat the oven to 425°F.

2. Place fish in an 11x7-inch baking dish coated with cooking spray.

3. Combine lime juice, mayonnaise, onion powder, and black pepper in a small bowl, and spread over fish.

4. Sprinkle with breadcrumbs; drizzle with Smart Start.

5. Bake for 20 minutes, or till the fish flakes easily while tested with a fork.

6. Sprinkle with parsley and serve.

Curried Baby Carrots

Ingredients

- 1⁄2 pound (4-inch) baby carrots

- 2 Tbsp. fat-free mayonnaise

- 1 Tbsp. nonfat sour cream

- 1⁄2 tsp. curry powder

- 1⁄2 tsp. skim milk

- 1⁄2 tsp. fresh lemon juice

- 1⁄2 tsp. honey

Instructions

1. Steam carrots, covered, 7 minutes or until crisp-tender; drain.

2. Combine mayonnaise and remaining ingredients in a saucepan; place over medium-low heat until hot, stirring occasionally.

3. Serve sauce with carrots.

Broke Bean Stew

Ingredients

- 1 Tbsp olive oil

- 1 large yellow or white onion, chopped

- 1 Tbsp chopped/minced garlic

- 1 tsp ground cumin

- 1 tsp chili powder

- 2 cans diced fire-roasted tomatoes (14.5oz)

- 3 cans (15.5 oz each) dark red kidney beans, black bean, white beans; rinsed & drained

- 4 cups fat-free low sodium chicken broth

- 1/4 cup chopped cilantro

- 3 cups fresh baby spinach leaves

Directions

1. Heat olive oil over medium-high heat in a 4-quart saucepan. Add onion and say about five minutes, until softened however not browned. Add garlic

and cook 1 minute longer. Do now no longer brown garlic.

2. Add spices and tomatoes and simmer for approximately five minutes. Add three cups (2 cans) of beans and a couple of cups of broth and bring to a boil. Reduce to a simmer.

three. Place remaining beans and broth in a bowl of a food processor or in a blender. Add cilantro and puree till smooth. Add mixture to stew. Add spinach and heat just till wilted. Stir well and serve hot.

Breakfast Burrito

Ingredients

- 3 large egg whites

- 1 strip nitrate-free turkey bacon, chopped

- 1/4 cup chopped onion

- 2 Tbsp. seeded, chopped fresh tomato

- 1 whole-wheat flour, 96% fat-free tortilla (8" diameter)

- 1/4 cup (1/2 ounce) finely shredded Cabot 75% Light Cheddar Cheese

- 2 tsp. red taco sauce

Instructions

1. Mist a small microwaveable bowl with olive oil spray. Add the egg whites. Set aside.

2. Set a small nonstick skillet over medium-excessive heat until it is hot enough for a spritz of water to sizzle on it. With an oven mitt, in short remove the pan from the heat to mist with cooking spray. Set over medium-high heat and upload the bacon. Cook, stirring occasionally, for about 2 minutes. Add the onion. Cook for 1 to two minutes, or until the bacon is crisp. Add the tomato. Cook for approximately 1 minute, or until just heated. Transfer the bacon mixture to a bowl. Cover to keep warm. Place the tortilla in the pan and go back to medium-high heat. Cook for about 30 seconds per side, or till just warm.

3. Meanwhile, microwave the egg whites on low power for 30 seconds. Continue microwaving in 30-second intervals until they are just a bit runny on top. Stir them with a fork, breaking into large pieces. If they are still undercooked, prepare dinner dinner them in 10-second intervals till just done. Stir in the reserved bacon mixture.

4. Place the tortilla on a serving plate. Sprinkle on the cheese leaving approximately 2" naked on one end, in an even strip (approximately 3" wide) running down the center. Top with the reserved egg white mixture and drizzle on the taco sauce. Fold the bare end of the tortilla up over the filling,

and then fold the edges of the tortilla over the middle. Serve your breakfast burrito immediately.

Summary

The Biggest Loser diet is a low calorie eating plan based on the reality tv show of the equal name.

It has been shown to aid weight loss by stressing meal planning, calorie counting, and portion control. Its meals are high fiber fruits, vegetables, and whole grains balanced with low fat proteins and small amounts of healthy fat.

Yet, it may dangerously restrict energy for some people and may be challenging to adhere to. What`s more, there`s no aid during or after the program to help you maintain weight loss.

Still, if you`re searching to consume healthful and

shed weight at the equal time, the Biggest Loser

diet may be worth a shot.